ENDORSEMENTS

"We have seen up close Susan's incredible life of enduring victoriously as her pastors and friends. As people who ourselves have personally known God as Jehovah Rapha, the Lord who heals, after a devastating health diagnosis, we encourage anyone who is facing their own hill of difficulty to read Susan's latest book, *I Beg To Differ*. Her story of faith, hope and healing will encourage you to look to God, His word and His character, as she shares her journey towards restoration and life."

Pastors Jonathan & Amy Kerridge
Gardn Church

"I was excited to read Susan's narrative of her journey to wholeness, and freedom in Christ. Yet the walk of faith in her God is a living testimony to the faithfulness of God to anyone who will dare to believe God means what His Word says, and hold steady through thick and thin, to Him and His promises. "A life transformed by the power of God, has become a beacon of hope to all who struggle with adversity in any form. This book is a must-read for those who need encouragement and desire to encourage others.

Thank you, Susan, for your transparency and courage but mostly for sharing your heart of love for God, and for others, through a life surrendered to His call. It is summed up in

Hebrews 11:6, "But without faith it is impossible to please and be satisfactory to Him. For whoever would come near God must believe that God exists and that He is the rewarder of those who earnestly and diligently seek Him."

Pastor Wendy Park
Restoration Ministries Australia
Wellington Point, Queensland

I BEG TO DIFFER

Susan Lambert

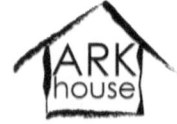

Ark House Press
arkhousepress.com

© 2025 Susan Lambert

All rights reserved. Apart from any fair dealing for the purpose of study, research, criticism, or review, as permitted under the Copyright Act, no part may be reproduced by any process without written permission.

Unless otherwise stated, all Scriptures are taken from the New International Translation (Holy Bible. Copyright© 1996, 2004, 2007, 2013 by Tyndale House Foundation. Used by permission of Tyndale House Publishers Inc., Carol Stream, Illinois 60188. All rights reserved.)

Some names and identifying details have been changed to protect the privacy of individuals.

Cataloguing in Publication Data:
Title: I Beg To Differ
ISBN: 978-1-7640542-4-9 (pbk)
Subjects: REL012170   RELIGION / Christian Living / Personal Memoirs;
Cover design by Eli Walker
Typeset by initiateagency.com

*To my husband, Greg,
My companion in Christ, my love and best friend.
Forever us.*

*To my sons, Jake and Clayton,
To be your mother has been the greatest
privilege and blessing of my life.*

*To my daughter-in-loves, Marissa and Brittany
Hand chosen by God to love our sons.
Forever grateful.*

*To my family and close friends who have prayed
and stood in faith with me over many years.*

CONTENTS

Endorsements.. i

Preface.. ix

1. The Waiting Room 1
2. Our Past Lingers 5
3. The Hill Of Difficulty 9
4. Yahweh Strengthens 13
5. Facing Our Fears 17
6. Finding Your Army 21
7. Choose Life 27
8. Understanding the Power of Hope 35
9. Adult Battles are not Children's Burdens 39
10. A Spiritual Sword 45
11. Restoration and Healing 49
12. Enduring Victoriously 53
13. Anguish in Your Soul 59
14. Let the Redeemed Tell Their Story 65

About the author 73

PREFACE

MY PREVIOUS SELF-PUBLISHED MEMOIR, *Dancing Daughter*, centered around a childhood amid family violence and my eventual path to a place of renewal, forgiveness, and healing.

I Beg to Differ has emerged under a quiet strengthening resolve to bring hope to those facing a life-threatening illness or adversity. One may have concluded from the end of my previous book that my new, shiny life was going to remain as a "happily ever after" tale.

The young naïve version of me had certainly hoped so.

But of course, I was to learn that life is not always as we expect it to be. It is an unfolding story that can "turn on a dime," a common phrase, my father so often used.

This book is about how my life did in fact *turn on a dime* at 38 years of age; a medical diagnosis that threatened to steal my brand-new life as a wife, and a mother of two young boys.

A medical diagnosis with an expiry date of three to five years was spoken over my life.

My brand-new life was forever changed one morning in a cold, sterile doctor's office.

This story is ultimately one of finding the courage to challenge the darkness of that diagnosis. The courage to come to know God as Jehovah Rapha, the Lord who heals in every aspect of our lives: physically, emotionally, and spiritually – because He alone is the mender of brokenness, the binder of all wounds.

And yet this story is about far more than standing in faith for a physical healing.

My story is a cautionary tale of sorts because it exposes how childhood trauma can influence and distort our view of who God really is.

Our view of God is significant in shaping ourselves and our relationship with Jesus.

My journey of seeking healing therefore, needed to initially confront a childhood narrative that was casting an inaccurate picture of who God really is.

How can we trust God and hold fast to His promises if we do not know Him intimately?

As C.S Lewis famously said, "I want God, not my idea of God."

The title of my book, *I Beg to Differ*, has been inspired by the following quote by an unnamed philosopher, rumoured to be a Celtic Christian early in the first century:

> *When I light a candle at midnight, I say to the darkness, I beg to differ.*

Midnight always seems to be the darkest of the night hours. Darkness in our life can arrive in many forms. It has been said that at some stage, we will all face *a dark night of the soul.*

A dark night of the soul that attempts to cast a taunting narrative, implying that we are hopeless, helpless, and alone.

PREFACE

Fear tries to declare that darkness is our whole story.

Faith in Jesus, however, lights a candle in that darkness and defiantly chooses to say:

I beg to differ.

God desires for each of us to hand our life story over to Him. Only then can we confidently say that every chapter of darkness that arrives in our lives, will be transformed into a story of courage, hope, and healing as we behold God in all His glory.

1 John 5 reminds us that whatever shadow of darkness has been cast upon our life, the light of Jesus will not be overwhelmed, and neither will you:

> "The light shines in the darkness, and the darkness
> has not overcome it."

At the time John wrote these words, when Jesus told his followers,

"You are the light of the world" there were no power grids, spot lights or flood lights.

There were just small flickering candle flames to light their world, vulnerable to being snuffed out.

Archbishop Desmond Tutu tells the powerful story of South African Christians placing lit candles in their windows to protest apartheid. So unsettling was their collective symbol of hope, the government passed a law making it illegal to light a candle and place it in your window.

Apartheid was eventually dismantled.

We are all called to be light in the world ___ again, and again, and again.

Our story, regardless of adversity is to reject the narrative of fear and darkness and reflect the light of the divine reality that can be found in Jesus.

We must be brave and place our candle in the window, and declare "I beg to differ"

How else will the world know that darkness does not have the final say?

CHAPTER 1

THE WAITING ROOM

I WAS SO ANGRY. I did not belong here. My life was just beginning.

I was only 38 years old, with a husband and two young sons to care for.

I purposefully chose to sit in a chair at the furthest reaches of the waiting room and defiantly crossed my arms. I sat in what I can only describe as an awkward unbelief.

I am ashamed to say I could barely look at the other patients in the waiting room, with their head scarves and grief-stricken, gaunt faces all screaming sickness at me.

Irrational fear whispered, *If you look at them, you might become one of them.*

The expressionless face of a young girl who was the receptionist did little to calm my anxiety as I watched her greet people with very little warmth. Life experience had mercifully not yet equipped her with the emotional empathy needed for the worried patients entering her world each day.

The waiting room was not overly crowded, although it still seemed oppressively small. The drab décor did little to lift the mood of the people waiting, with its beige carpet and out-dated, uncomfortable brown arm chairs.

The doctor suddenly appeared in the framed doorway of his office and called my name, and I am not sure if it was something in the tone of his voice, or the way he averted his eyes from mine, but fear gripped me in the depths of my being.

I suddenly hated the way I had this strange ability to always discern danger.

No doubt my hyper-vigilant nature was possibly a by-product of a childhood spent navigating an alcoholic father.

We were ushered into the specialist's room and what I recall most was the breathtaking view. Wide glass windows ran sweepingly along one wall and almost allowed the sky to reach into the room and touch us.

My husband reached for my hand as the doctor sat and swiveled in his black leather chair for a few minutes, reading his notes. The large polished dark wood table placed an immediate barrier between us, and I remember feeling a sense of powerlessness.

He starting nervously shuffling pieces of paper, and with limited eye contact and barely any emotion, he spoke the words that would change the trajectory of my life forever.

"You have a type of blood cancer. It is called Multiple Myeloma."

Adrenaline coursed through my body and shock had me leaping out of the chair straight to the window to catch a glimpse of the outside world. I was desperately trying to normalise the situation and regulate my emotions.

The blue sky and the ocean seemed to taunt me, so contrasting in beauty were they to this shattering diagnosis. I could hear a firm voice from behind me.

"Come and sit down please."

The doctor seemed out of his depth with a patient who had reacted with such emotional intensity; an emotional intensity that was quite possibly the by-product of a fearful childhood.

A by product that made the young child in me, suddenly feel completely powerless.

I walked slowly and somewhat defiantly back to my chair, sat down, and folded my arms to try and protect myself.

On reflection, I was unfairly rude to this specialist, who no doubt needed boundaries to preserve himself, such was the nature of his work each day. It still, however, troubles me, the lack of empathy and the stark, cold settings in which life-changing medical results are sometimes handed to patients.

He continued with more information to try and exert some semblance of control over the situation.

"It is a slow-moving cancer and there are treatments that we can use to try and slow its progress. It is however, incurable."

He spoke as if the extra information was somehow meant to soften the initial blow. It did nothing to allay the sickening fear that was slowly building up inside of me.

Layer, upon layer, upon layer of fear. You know the type: the type that takes hold deep inside your gut and drains every ounce of strength from you. The type that leaves your mouth dry and your heart thumping in your chest.

"No cure?" my husband questioned again. I suspect he was hoping for a different answer.

My husband squeezed my hand a little tighter as I sat motionless and stared at the far wall and he asked the bravest of questions.

"What is the prognosis?"

The doctor paused, perhaps contemplating the professional wisdom of even answering his question.

Three to five years.

It was like a court room judge had just dropped his gavel and delivered a death sentence.

CHAPTER 2

OUR PAST LINGERS

SHOCK IS AN UNFORGIVING, brutal place to be. It can transport you back to places you never want to go again. Places from your past. Places you mistakenly thought you had left behind.

Suddenly, I found myself there again.

I was that seven-year-old girl, crouched in the corner of the back verandah of my childhood home, covering my ears to dull the shouting of a drunken father, hands clasped together, praying, and crying out to God for a miracle. Tears running down my face as I begged God to make the yelling stop. That same, familiar terror had suddenly and unexpectedly arrived in my life again.

The same sense of utter hopelessness.

I thought I had finally moved into a safe, calm, predictable place in my life. Things were finally coming together after I had spent a childhood waiting for the danger to pass.

I was married to a man that was everything my father had failed to be, and we had two beautiful boys. Things were finally looking up. I was beginning to trust in the goodness of God a little.

Shock had me trapped in a daze as we left the doctor's office. I cannot even remember the drive home with my husband. I do remember running straight to my bedroom and crawling under the covers of our bed. Shock felt like a bitter, almost evil coldness rolling over my body, that no number of blankets could seem to alleviate. The waves of grief were relentless.

It was the grief of a mother who was going to be torn away from her family by a disease that she felt she had no control over. We told our sons I had the flu to cover for my disconnectedness.

My husband continued with the same amazing consistency that he has always approached our marriage and fatherhood with; a consistency that remains the greatest gift a wife and family could ask for.

Especially this wife, who had endured a childhood filled with inconsistency. I never knew what version of my father would greet our family at the end of the day. Sadly, most days, he was the violent, drunken, lesser version of himself, a version that was silently shaping my view of men, and of greater significance, my view of God.

A false narrative was building in the background of my life.

God was not consistently faithful.

Of course, I did not realise this at the time. The false narrative was like a silent melody playing subtle notes in the background of my life. It would take some sad, lost years after I left home before I started to challenge that destructive narrative.

My husband was a large part of disrupting and changing my inaccurate view of God with his dependable nature. God had no doubt given me a husband of consistency because He knew exactly what the broken little girl inside me needed.

And yet, if you are reading this story as a single person, know that it was not my husband who saved me. God may have used the attributes of my husband to challenge my destructive childhood narrative, but there is only One who can truly save and heal.

That one is Jesus.

He alone, is the way, the truth, and the life.

He is an intimate, personal, loving Father, waiting for you to surrender your life to Him.

The tentacles of victimhood can be subtle and somewhat alluring.

We can stay in our fear because it starts to feel familiar, and in some strange way, it seems to lure us and promise a false sense of safety.

CHAPTER 3

THE HILL OF DIFFICULTY

IN LIFE, YOU HAVE probably worked out by now that there will be some really hard things: storms to weather, mountains to confront, sadnesses to bear. We should not be surprised, as we are told this by Jesus himself.

And yet, my young, naïve heart was surprised.

This was not the life I thought I would have, nor the life I wanted, a life navigating a serious health challenge.

> *"But I have told you these things, so that in me you*
> *may have peace.*
> *In this world you will have trouble.*
> *But take heart! I have overcome the world."*
> *(John 16:33)*

Take heart?

Take heart in biblical Hebrew translates as "strengthen your heart" or "take courage."

What does that even mean in a situation that seems un-winnable? Take heart for me, at first, simply meant finding the strength to get off my bed. Deep down, I knew a choice was standing between me and any semblance of a future.

Two paths were beckoning; two ways I could respond: the way of faith, or the way of fear.

One of survivor, or one of victim.

One of living in the darkness of the diagnosis, or walking in the light.

I recall walking out to the lounge room of our home for the first time after a whole day of pretending to be bed-bound by flu. What struck me so profoundly was our two lively, energetic boys as they rushed past me toward the back garden to play.

"Feeling better, Mummy?" they asked.

A childlike optimism, not yet dimmed by the world, filled their sparkling, expectant eyes. The abandonment of childhood beamed back at me as they ran past me on their way to somewhere else.

Watching them play together in the warm sunshine, free from fear, only served to strengthen my resolve.

John Bunyan, in his novel, The Pilgrims Progress, captured the beckoning of the two different ways I could respond to my diagnosis:

> *There were also in the same place two other ways*
> *besides that which came straight from the gate;*
>   *Often appearing the hardest of ways.*

> *One turned to the left hand, and the other to the right, at the bottom of the hill: but the narrow way lay right up the hill.*
>
> *This hill though high, I covet to ascend;*
> *The difficulty will not me offend,*
> *For I perceive the way to life lays here:*
> *Come, pluck up, heart, lets neither faint nor fear!*
> *Better, though difficult, the right way to go,*
> *Then wrong, though easy, where the end is woe.*

Plucking up heart, as suggested by Bunyan, is easier said than done and it sounds a lot like the "take heart" posture Jesus speaks of.

Sometimes, the seemingly easier way in life can look enticing at first. We can stay in our fear and it feels familiar, and in some strange way, it seems to lure us and promise a place of safety.

The tentacles of victimhood can be subtle and somewhat alluring.

Just stay here, this is too hard to handle, way too much to bear. Just stay, sitting in your pain.

Now I am not advocating that we cannot sit and feel our pain. It is important to process our grief and it takes different amounts of time for each of us.

What I am advocating is what I have found to be true in my own life. Remaining in that pain as a victim to our circumstances for too long steals way too much from us. It steals our hope, and inevitably, it can steal any semblance of a future, whatever that may look like. If I had adopted a victim's identity it would have looked something like this:

A young wife and mother of two young boys with an incurable disease, with an end date determined by a medical prognosis based on statistics. Only God knows our end date. The day we leave this earth is determined by Him.

Despite my diagnosis, I chose God's prognosis.

So, with very little courage and a God that I thought had abandoned me as a young child, I chose to step out of being a victim. This time I would not stay crouched in fear in the corner of the verandah of my childhood home.

This time, I would search for the true character of God according to His word, not a version of Him, tainted by my childhood wounds. A version of God that was based on biblical truth and a personal knowledge of Him, not one based upon my life circumstances.

I would choose the narrow way, straight up the face of the mountain that stood squarely in front of me.

The mountain that I had been told by doctors was impossible to climb.

CHAPTER 4

YAHWEH STRENGTHENS

Growing up in a conservative Anglican church with incense, organ-grinding hymns and the Bible read only by the priest in robes every Sunday, shaped my early view of God. And while none of these expressions of faith were necessarily wrong, and I was blessed to be introduced to God there, it had not given me the power I needed to change my life.

It was like I knew all these things about God, but had not yet actually encountered Him for myself. My diagnosis forced me to look squarely at the character of God.

Not a view of God informed by spiritual immaturity, childhood trauma or merely an intellectual grasp of theology, but rather a view formed from a real and brave journey of desperation, a place of needing to meet God face to face. I needed to find a personal God, a God who understood my pain, my deep sadness, and my fear for the future.

Personal desperation is quite often the very place that God meets with us.

One night, after the children were in bed, I sat and cried, as I had done many nights before.

Because we had not yet chosen to burden the children with my diagnosis, long days holding in my grief would sometimes overflow in the evenings. One night, I was crying and searching through my Bible for a glimmer of hope in a seemingly hopeless situation. It was then I stumbled across the writings of Hezekiah, King of Judah in the book of Isaiah.

Nothing could prepare me for what I was about to read. The similarities to my own situation were beyond striking. Hezekiah had written about his deepest grief due to a serious illness.

As I read, I wept.

Hezekiah had screamed the same angry questions at God that I had.

> *In the prime of my life*
> *must I go through the gates of death*
> *and be robbed of the rest of my years?"*
> *I will not again see the Lord, in the land of the living?*
> *No longer will I look on mankind,*
> *Or be with those who now dwell in this world.*
> *(Isaiah 38: 10, 11)*

And he described the same relentless grief I was feeling.

> *I cried like a swift or thrush,*
> *I moaned like a mourning dove.*
> *My eyes grew weak as I looked to the heavens.*

YAHWEH STRENGTHENS

I am troubled; O Lord, come to my aid!
(Isaiah 38 :14,15)

That night, I felt like God had seen me.

He saw my fears and my desperation. The story of Hezekiah reached in and somehow touched my spirit in a way that is difficult to articulate. Of course, I understand the importance of reading scripture through the lens of historical context, but somewhere, deep in my spirit, something of the miraculous side of God was sown.

If God could hear Hezekiah's prayer and restore him to health, perhaps he could do that for me.

Hope stirred.

The power of sharing our story of faith can never be underestimated. Our story, just like Hezekiah's, can change lives. God is always searching for the brave among us, willing to be vulnerable with our struggles. Imagine if Hezekiah had not chosen to write about those real and raw questions he asked of God?

How many people have stumbled across his writings, just as I have, and related to his grief, and more importantly, been encouraged to cry out to God with their real feelings?

Of greater significance is the strength and hope for the future his story imparts to others.

The name Hezekiah in the Hebrew translates as "Yahweh strengthens."

That night as I closed my Bible, I felt strengthened indeed.

And now that depth of childhood fear, that had been silently waiting in the wings of my adult life, had found an opportunity to take centre stage again.

CHAPTER 5

FACING OUR FEARS

As FOLLOWERS OF JESUS, I believe we are all called to be messengers of hope and healing in a broken world.

Over the coming days we shared my diagnosis with only a handful of very close friends and family, those we trusted to be confidential. All reacted differently. Some rose in faith. Some ran scared. Some broke our confidentiality and told others.

And yet, in the end, regardless of how other people reacted to my diagnosis, the truth for me was slowly becoming a far more daunting prospect. Other people's reactions, opinions, theological views on faith and healing, or even their empathy were not going to save me.

I knew I had to mature in my understanding of faith and my personal relationship with God. It was becoming abundantly clear: my immature view of a God was no match for the spiritual battle I had unexpectedly found myself in. My expectation that He would keep me safe in a protected cocoon had been burst wide open in spectacular fashion. I naïvely thought it meant I would be protected from all the hard things in life ever again.

I started throwing angry protests at God, bargaining with Him.

I reminded him of how awful my childhood was. Had I not earned some happiness now? Could I please just have a little longer on this mountain top with my husband and two beautiful boys before plummeting me into another valley? I was like an angry little girl, stomping her feet.

I did not want to be in this valley. It was way too dark.

I was always afraid of the dark growing up.

I almost feel ashamed to say that this fear was still with me well into my late teens.

I suspect the fear was entrenched from having to escape to safety in the back seat of our family car in the middle of the night.

Nights were always the hardest in my childhood home. A place that should have been a refuge of safety often became a place of terror. Terror might seem like a strong word to use, but that is the depth of fear that used to grip me as a young child. Late at night, my father would be at his drunkest and his physical aggression would always be slowly building.

My mother always knew when it was time. Time to leave.

Fleeing to the car with her was always a secret mission, performed quietly with hushed tones so as not to alert my father. I was delegated to the back seat with my sister, while my older brother rode up front. Back in those days, we all had to lock our doors individually, so the sound of those four separate clicks became a moment of great relief as we drove away, and we were safely locked in the cocoon of the car.

And now, that depth of childhood fear, that had been silently waiting in the wings of my adult life, had found an opportunity to take centre stage again.

The main fear that cast the blackest of shadows over me was a brutal one. It is a fear that my heart wishes no young mother should ever have to confront.

The fear of death.

The fear of leaving my young children.

Fear of death is a formidable opponent; an opponent that can gate crash our lives unfairly and unexpectedly.

I would like to tell you that God helped me conquer my fear immediately, but for me, that was not what happened. If you are reading this and you are facing a health battle that is life threatening, I know you will immediately understand the fear that can take hold deep in your inmost being.

What I am about to say is so very hard, but I believe it is a place we must allow ourselves to go, if we are to find real freedom from fear, as we walk out our journey toward healing and wholeness.

We must face our own mortality.

At the beginning of our battle, we must bravely stare down our gravest of fears.

Facing our own mortality is such an overwhelming and courageous stance, but ultimately, I believe it is a crucial part of our healing journey with God.

Facing our mortality with God beside us, is not a position of defeat, nor is it a lack of faith.

It is not a position of giving up, or not contending for the promises that can be found in the word of God.

In fact, I believe it is quite the opposite. I believe facing our own mortality disarms the enemy of his fiercest weapon.

The weapon of fear.

> *Even when your path takes me through the valley of deepest darkness,*
> *Fear will never conquer me, for you already have!*
> *Your authority is my strength and my peace.*
> *The comfort of your love takes away my fear.*
> *(Psalm 23 v 4 TPT version)*

CHAPTER 6

FINDING YOUR ARMY

GOD WAS NOT SHOCKED by my diagnosis of cancer. He knew the path that lay ahead.

> *I will go before you and make the rough places smooth. (Isaiah 45.2)*

I understand this scripture refers to God making a way for the Assyrian exiles returning to Israel. However, it would soon become obvious that He had also been preparing a way for me too. God had begun to mobilise His troops long before I found myself in that doctor's office… troops to help me stand up on my feet.

No doubt there was going to be some challenging spiritual combat ahead, and I needed to be equipped and learn from those who had been to battle before. The battles we have already weathered, and the rough places God has made smooth for us, holds precious wisdom for others.

Those battles are meant to be the substance of our faith journey.

A faith journey that holds hard fought wisdom for others.

1 Peter 3:15 holds a powerful message regarding this:

Always be prepared to give an answer to everyone who asks you the reason for the hope that you have.

I urge you as a Christian to always be prepared to offer hope to those who cross your path.

One of those people was me. A young married wife and mother who needed to hear the hope found in God's word. Be brave and step into the battle with others. Be part of believing and standing beside those in your world that need to anchor their hope in Jesus.

The first few weeks, I was literally inundated with fellow believers who would randomly cross my path wherever I found myself. Dropping the boys to school, at the supermarket, the hairdresser, a women's lunch at church. These people did not know my diagnosis, and yet, they felt prompted to share their story. One after another, during conversation, their stories all had one incredible truth in common.

God had healed their cancer or held their life-threatening disease for unexpectedly long periods of time.

I am the Lord that heals thee had become part of their faith story.

This was so very challenging for me. Perhaps these Christians had more faith than me? Perhaps they were super-spiritual? Perhaps they had some special call or purpose on their lives?

I am being real here. I was just a girl from the country, a young mother with a couple of kids, a new Christian at that, who found herself needing to be healed.

Does God even do the extraordinary in the ordinary lives of people?

I thought healing must have been reserved for those chosen ones.

And perhaps the most challenging theological question of all confronted me:

Was God still healing people today?

And if so, who was I to think I would see a miracle of healing in my own life?

My entire childhood had been spent praying and begging God to turn up and rescue me. The child in me thought He never came. My father remained an alcoholic until I left home, bound for university. Why would He come now, the little girl in me reasoned?

I felt abandoned by God, even though He had been with me my entire life.

At this point in my story, I need to pause.

I have to say how hard this story has been to write. I have stopped writing, time and time again. I am not sharing my faith story in any way to diminish yours.

I am writing my story, to bring hope to you.

If you are reading this and someone you loved dearly is no longer on earth, I am so sorry for your loss. I understand, completely. My own mother and sister-in-law were not healed earthside. I am therefore not oblivious to pain and loss, nor am I naïve about the spiritual battle that rages around us.

I understand we live in a broken world.

As Christians, we must be allowed to say that we do not always understand the mystery that is healing. There will be times in our life when we will all experience spiritual doubts and confusion; times when we are called to stand firm in faith, believing what Jesus said to be true, even when we do not fully understand.

Why are some healed on earth and others when they are heaven-side?

God will always elude our finite rational understanding. The facts of this broken world are all around us, hemming us in, with overwhelming intensity at times.

Sometimes, that brokenness touches our lives or those closest to us, in tragic ways. I never want to minimise or deny anyone's pain.

As I am writing this book, two of my friends are each battling a serious cancer diagnosis, but my friends' battles have only served to strengthen my resolve to write my story. I am, however, passionate about writing my story with authenticity and empathy, but most importantly, with the utmost respect for the truth of God's Word and His character. In all honesty, as I wrote, the world seemed to get darker.

The spiritual battle we are all in, seemed to be more illuminated than ever.

BUT... the facts of this broken world will ALWAYS oppose Gods truth.

And a spiritual battle needs a spiritual response.

And that spiritual response must be the living, active, powerful word of Gods truth.

It is our living hope. The hope of Christ in us.

Let us hold unswervingly to the hope we professed for He who promised is faithful. (Heb 10.23)

My deepest desire is to reveal the light of God that only He can bring to those who may be facing the darkest of days.

Even in darkness light dawns for the upright. (Psalm 112.4)

It is to encourage you to live HEALED, despite your diagnosis.

I know that may sound strange... counterintuitive almost. How does one live healed when they are sick? How does one live healed when they are depressed? How does one live healed when they are anxious?

This is not a denial of our circumstances. It is the choice to pursue and lean into the supernatural power of Jesus available to each one of us.

Bear with me, as I share a little more of my story, the part where God helped me understand some truths about Jesus and the depth of his love for us.

A love so powerful that it helped me find a way to rise above my circumstances, as I sought to live in the abundant, whole life, Jesus came to bring to each of us.

The part where God helped me decide once and for all, to light a candle and defiantly place it right in the middle of the overwhelming darkness cast upon me from a life-threatening disease.

Faith is an ongoing,
transformative
wrestle with God.

We grow spiritually only
to the extent we allow
Him access to our life.

CHAPTER 7

CHOOSE LIFE

I WANT MY STORY to share the real and authentic path I walked as I was seeking to understand the healing power of God. I want to share with you all the aspects of faith I personally had to wrestle with.

Faith is an ongoing, transformative wrestle with God, as we allow Him access to our life.

The greatest challenge as a Christian, at least for me personally, was how do I reconcile my faith in God with the hard facts of my broken circumstances? Are we to abandon our rational, intellectual thoughts altogether? Not at all.

We are however, called to bring faith and rational thought into proper relationship.

Oswald Chambers, in his devotional *My Utmost for His Highest*, captures the reconciliation needed for those of us who are learning to live by faith.

Faith in active opposition to common sense is mistaken enthusiasm and narrow mindedness, and common sense in opposition to faith demonstrates a mistaken reliance on reason as the basis of truth. The life of faith brings the two of these into proper relationship.

The important truth here is not to abandon one for the other.

There is a place for intellectual, rational, common sense in our healing journey. God can use every resource available to bring healing to you. Of course, you need to pray and seek God in your decision making around medical intervention.

I personally have chosen not to abandon my intellectual rational thought on my healing journey.

Medical science and faith can co-exist together.

I personally know of a growing number of people who have experienced miraculous responses to cancer with the new treatment of immunotherapy.

It is the reason I have a blood test every year, and choose to see my specialist, who has expertise in blood cancer. The blood test has, in fact, become the rational evidence that has only served to reveal to me, the healing Hand of God, holding back my disease.

God has used the rational evidence to make His perfect faith real to me.

Chambers speaks of this:

> *For every detail of common sense in life, there is a truth God has revealed by which we can prove in our practical experience, what we believe God to be.*

God is personal and our faith journey is the outworking of our relationship with Him.

Our experience of God, what we know to be true in our own life, becomes the substance of our faith.

"The transforming power of God's providence transforms perfect faith into reality. Faith always works in a personal way because the purpose of God is to see that perfect faith is made real in His children.

As we experience and see the miraculous Hand of God in our own lives, His perfect faith is indeed made real to each of us.

I also feel it is important to speak about the importance of our emotional health when we are facing adversity of any kind. Denying how we really feel as an expression of strong faith is not biblical, nor is it a healthy response. Disregarding how we feel is not what God expects us to do.

The notion that strong faith is devoid of emotion is simply not true. I believe it is what God asks us to do with those emotions, however, which is an important part of learning how to walk by faith in Him.

Cast your cares upon him, because he cares for you. (1 Peter 5)

To cast means the intentional action of laying our burdens and anxieties on the Lord.

How do we cast our cares?

Every time we feel overwhelmed by feelings of defeat, share all your sadness with the Lord. Every time, He promises to meet us there, right in the middle of the mess.

Every time doubts of His goodness try to creep into our thinking, lay those doubts quickly at His feet.

Every time, God will overcome those doubts by strengthening our faith in Him.

Our feelings are of great significance to God. Bring them all to Him.

But I have digressed, so let us return to my story because I am eager to share with you one of the most significant and foundational steps one must adopt.

At first, this may sound almost too simplistic to be of any help. However, it has proven to be perhaps the most profound and sustaining decision I made.

It was to make a choice. A brave choice.

A choice to choose LIFE.

To choose a place of victory, despite my diagnosis.

In the beginning, it was other believers who stood beside me and helped me make my choice. I was feeling way too discouraged in the beginning to even pray. It was other believers who dared to speak hope and life to me that gradually began to build my spiritual bravery, while my doubts and the medical diagnosis in the natural were screaming fear.

I could strongly sense God nudging me to understand the power of making a choice.

The choice to choose life.

A choice that said, "Lord, I will fix my gaze upon You."

Let Deuteronomy 30:9 become your unwavering foundation.

This day I call heaven and earth as witnesses against you that I have set before you, life and death, blessings, and curses. Now choose life, so that you and your children may live and that you may love the Lord your God, listen to his voice, and hold fast to Him.

I suspect I know what you are thinking at this point. This all sounds very encouraging, BUT... you cannot see the size of this mountain overshadowing my life.

How can I choose life when this diagnosis is so dark? How can I choose life when the doctors have spoken such negativity over my future?

It is because choosing life is far more powerful than we can fully comprehend.

Choosing life, is choosing to fix our gaze on Jesus.

Choosing life is choosing God's Word above our circumstances.

Choosing life is choosing to live by faith and not by fear.

So, faith cometh by hearing, and hearing by the word of God (Romans 10:17)

I have also come to understand that it is not enough to know the word of God intellectually. We must meditate on it, so it becomes living and active on the inside of us.

For the word of God is alive and powerful. It is sharper than the sharpest two-edged sword. (Hebrews 4:12)

This is not a demanding posture of faith, and nor is it an arrogant, misguided belief that if I say it, it will happen.

It is simply a posture of faith that defiantly declares I am choosing to dwell on healing, rather than sickness.

Start by speaking the healing word of God out loud and quietly under your breath, whenever fear and anxiety comes into your mind.

Replace every anxious thought with God's word.

If I am brutally honest, I did not even believe what I was saying at first. The diagnosis was far too loud and far too scary; a diagnosis so loud that in the beginning it drowned out those scriptures.

But I said them anyway.

I choose life in Jesus' name.

An illness with no cure was clearly not the best of odds.

Thank you, Jesus, that by your stripes I am healed and made whole. (Isaiah 53:5)

Other people will say I am in denial.

The Lord restores my health and heals my wounds. (Jeremiah 30:17)

I carried those scriptures everywhere. I had a little book small enough to fit in my pocket with all the healing scriptures I needed. The little book full of healing scriptures became my strength as I went about my day.

I was slowly renewing my mind.

Medical science aids healing through physical means by administering medicine into the physical body. God's Divine Healing is spiritual. It is administered through the human spirit.

Even medical science supports the importance of our words and their effect on our immune system. Numerous research findings suggest that people who have an image of themselves in poor health seem to confess that poor health and live out that reality, even if they are in fact in good health.

How much greater and more powerful is speaking God's word and creating an image of health and wholeness in our lives?

God has much to say about the power of His word.

> *My son, attend to my words; incline thine ear unto my sayings.*
> *Let them not depart from thine eyes; keep them amid thine heart.*

For they are life unto those that find them, and health to all their flesh. (Proverbs 4:20-22).

I kept reading and meditating on those healing words from God. It is hard to articulate, but ever so slowly, something began to slowly change. Deep inside, something was being planted. The spiritual part of me, my inmost being was growing stronger.

It was not optimism, nor was it positive thinking.

It was faith. Biblical faith.

"I pray that from his glorious riches he may strengthen you with power through his Spirit in your inner being." (Eph 3:16)

Hope is not an elusive, abstract concept.

Hope in God is the confident expectation that the goodness of God remains unchanged, regardless of our life circumstances.

CHAPTER 8

UNDERSTANDING THE POWER OF HOPE

THE NEXT SPIRITUAL KEY on my healing journey was the significance of fully understanding the power of God that is woven into Hope.

Hope is not an elusive, abstract concept.

Hope in God is the confident expectation that the goodness of God remains unchanged regardless of your circumstances.

It is not worldly hope or false hope; it is a living hope the Bible speaks of.

It is a settled confidence in God's character and His ability to fulfil what He has promised.

Hopelessness can be debilitating.

Adversity and sickness can steal our hope.

Without hope, we have nothing.

Hope deferred makes the heart sick, but a longing fulfilled is a tree of life. (Proverbs 13:2)

The Hebrew word for "hope" in the Bible is "Tikvah".

This word comes from the root, which means to twist strands of rope together to make a tool capable of holding a heavy load securely. This *rope of hope* is made stronger when we weave it together with others. You were not designed to hold onto this hope in God alone.

The enemy uses adversity to try and isolate us, and this diminishes the power of God in your life. Bravely reach out to those around you, even when you do not feel like it.

Again, truly I tell you if two of you agree on earth about anything they ask for, it will be done for them by my Father in heaven. For where two or three gather in my name, there I am with them. (Matthew 18: 19-20)

Every person standing with you in prayer and support as you face your mountain of adversity becomes another strand in your hope rope.

We have this hope as an anchor for the soul, firm and secure. It enters the inner sanctuary behind the curtain, where Jesus has entered on our behalf. (Hebrews 6:19, 20)

We cannot conjure up hope in our own strength. It is not an act of our own will. God pours hope into us through the power of the Holy Spirit.

Hopelessness is what had accompanied me my whole childhood, always hoping for my father to change and for our family to finally feel safe. A childhood spent in never-ending cycles of hope and despair.

Hope that he would overcome his addiction to alcohol, followed by disappointment, time and time again. A growing sense that nothing in life could change slowly took hold of me as a young girl.

A deep core belief that overcoming difficulty was almost impossible.

We are often unaware of how our childhood wounds can continue to bleed into our adult lives. Those wounds may even lay dormant, until something significant in our life opens them up again. Changes and transitions in our life such as becoming a parent, unexpected grief, or in my case, a health crisis, had awakened those fears.

If we ignore our past wounds and think they will just disappear, there is a real risk our lives will be built upon deception.

A subtle deception that communicates falsehoods about ourselves, but of greater significance, the true character of God.

Falsehoods that may become stumbling blocks to the abundant, whole, healed life God desires for each of us. It is a hard battle to confront our past wounds, and yet it is a critical part of our path to transformation and restoration.

The young girl in me had to challenge the destructive lies I had inherited from my childhood.

Is God faithful, and can I place my hope in Him?

My childhood had been stolen by fear and I was not about to watch history repeat itself in my family.

Faith not fear would define us, regardless of the outcome.

CHAPTER 9

ADULT BATTLES ARE NOT CHILDREN'S BURDENS

BECOMING A PARENT WAS one of the greatest gifts of my life. We had been blessed with two sons, and they were aged six and four years at the time of my diagnosis. The enormity of the decision of whether to tell our children about the health battle we faced, sat heavily on both my husband and I.

They were so very young. So very innocent. So very untouched by the world.

As an early childhood educator, I knew what the wisdom of the world professed.

It went something like this:

Be completely open with your children. Tell them everything.

Be transparent, otherwise, you will break your trust relationship with them.

Breaking our trust relationship with our children was of grave concern to us as parents.

One of our strongest core family values was based around honesty with each other.

At first, it seemed so contradictory not to tell them about my health diagnosis. Especially when I have a personality that leans toward openness and transparency with others… an openness God had used in my life to help others.

But what was God's wisdom in this situation?

James reminds us:

> *If any of you lacks wisdom, you should ask God, who gives generously to all without finding fault, and it will be given to you. (James 1 v5)*

We prayed and paused, and waited on His guidance. My specialist had given us three months until the next follow up blood test, as he had adopted a wait-and-see approach. We had some time, and so we decided initially to keep the diagnosis to ourselves.

God gave us the supernatural strength to rise in faith and continue as parents to our beautiful sons, as normally as we could.

The lioness in this mother had slowly been awakened and I was becoming increasingly determined to protect our boys at any cost. My childhood had been stolen by trauma and fear and I was not about to watch history repeat itself in my family.

I did not want illness to define our family.

Faith, not fear, would define us, regardless of the outcome.

Fear was not going to derail the purposes and plans God had established for my sons' lives.

ADULT BATTLES ARE NOT CHILDREN'S BURDENS

I think sometimes we can over-complicate God's guidance in our decision making and the overall direction of our lives. We can overthink and over-analyze His leadings. Can I encourage you to learn to just wait. God will give you a sense of peace as you make decisions and move through your life. We may never fully and confidently grasp His leadings.

Moving through is the key.

He is not controlling or prescriptive, nor does He limit your freedom to choose. The Bible, however, is meant to guide our decisions; decisions based upon the truth of God's Word.

He desires to bless you with the most abundant future possible as you keep Him at the centre of your life.

> *I know the plans I have for you, declares the Lord:*
> *Plans to prosper you and not to harm you,*
> *Plans to give you a hope and a future. (Jeremiah 29:11.)*

My husband and I prayed together and separately about the decision to tell our boys.

Over the next three months, we would share what each of us was sensing. We did not feel the need to rush such a huge decision. The way of the world is chaotic, loud, and rushed. It pushes us to make decisions in haste; decisions we may later regret. This decision had far-reaching consequences for our family.

We were learning the importance of pausing before we made the big decisions.

Sometimes the fear of deciding keeps many of us paralysed. Me included.

We must be brave enough to step out, decide, and set our God-given course.

From a place of humility, we must understand that of course all our decisions will not be perfect, but ultimately, decisions must be made.

A pause is not meant to be a long-term strategy.

I had grown up carrying adult burdens and fighting battles I was never meant to be in.

I personally knew the role reversal that sometimes happens in a childhood of chaos and trauma, and it does not play out well for children when they become adults.

In a house with an alcoholic father, I was often carrying the burden of the role of peacemaker in our home. I was on high alert to discern the mood and level of drunkenness of my father when he arrived home, and then be ready to act accordingly.

There were many long nights spent ballroom dancing with him to distract his attention away from my mother, to protect her from his physical abuse.

There was no doubt that my own childhood was also influencing my decision to carry the emotional burden of the diagnosis myself.

God works like that.

ADULT BATTLES ARE NOT CHILDREN'S BURDENS

He takes the hard parts of our lives and somehow turns them for good, if we allow Him.

In my case, a front row seat as a child living in fear gave me first-hand knowledge of what I did not want for my children.

Our decision was ultimately made with the same strong conviction from both of us.

There was to be no laying adult burdens upon our young boys. I desperately wanted our children to remain children, free to play and run and laugh with abandonment.

Free from the unbridled fear of losing their mother.

Children were not designed to carry adult burdens.

The weight of the world would come soon enough.

God was gently nudging me
to lay down my childhood
sword of survival and
take up a spiritual one.

CHAPTER 10

A SPIRITUAL SWORD

AS A CHILD, I was always on guard. Sword raised high. Watching and waiting. A childhood spent on high alert. Listening acutely for any signs of trouble. Listening for my father's arrival home. A slammed back door became my warning signal, a call to arms of sort.

And here I was again, a fully grown woman, feeling like another back door had been violently slammed.

The little girl inside me had lurched to attention, and I grabbed for that old familiar childhood sword to defend myself. And while that may have served me well as a child who was living in survival mode, it would soon become clear that it was a stance that I could not possibly sustain as an adult.

A stance that made me think I was in control of everything, that the battle would be won or lost by me.

It was an exhausting posture. The sword was getting far too heavy.

God was gently nudging me to lay down my childhood sword and take up a spiritual one.

My new strength had to come from an inner place, a place of trust, a place of handing the outcome over to God. A place that was sustainable. Handing the outcome over to God seemed like an impossible task for me.

I mean, this was not just some minor outcome. This outcome had dire, scary, life-threatening consequences. This outcome was everything to me. The process of handing the outcome over to God was a long and hard-fought battle for me.

If I am honest, it is a battle that at times, still rages to this day.

How do we face our battle, and yet leave the outcome to Him?

In reminding ourselves of victories past. In daily surrender.

I trust you Lord, with my life, whispered from the depths of our spirit.

Healing and transformation can look different for each of us.

We are individual people, with individual needs, and personal paths to tread as we seek healing from God. If you are facing a chronic health battle, as with many things in personal discipleship, there is no one-size-fits-all approach.

There is only the truth of His word and the power of the Holy spirit, as we walk out our personal faith journeys. Sometimes we can feel discouraged if we do not get a spontaneous healing right up front. This was the case for me.

I was scheduled to return to my doctor in three months' time. In the interim, I had met more Christians who shared with me that they had experienced a physical healing from God.

I went to healing services and several Christians laid hands on me and prayed. I fasted and detoxed my body from all sugar and processed food and was on a very specific diet from a naturopath. I sat in that doctor's office three months later, anticipating more positive news.

"Mrs Lambert, your blood test shows your marker for myeloma has risen slightly, but it is still in the stable range."

I walked out of the doctor's office feeling really defeated.

But I continued. I continued because of who God was.

God's healing word literally became the mainstay of my days and weeks. I maintained my new health regime without wavering. Then, six months later, the same result. 12 months later, same result. The myeloma cells were still showing in my blood test and other markers were clearly indicating its presence. I was starting to feel tired from the constant battle I found myself in.

The right food, the right exercise, the right immune-boosting vitamins, and the right prayers.

Now I am not saying all these lifestyle changes did nothing. Of course, they helped my body and God will often give us wisdom and keys to physical healing.

What I am saying is that somewhere along the way, there had been a very subtle shift in my faith that began to whisper:

I can heal thyself.

There is a very fine line between the belief that my faith can heal me, or my faith in God can heal me.

I thought if I stopped any of the daily health rituals that I had embraced, my cancer would become active. Fear and anxiety started to return because I thought I was in control of the outcome.

I was moving into works-based faith, relying on my own efforts for God's intervention.

The Apostle Paul, warns us of this subtle shift in our faith.

That if it is by grace, then it is no longer by works; otherwise, grace is no longer grace.

(Romans 11:6.)

The anointing of healing is purely and utterly by the grace and mercy found in God alone.

Faith is a gift from a loving God.

I was mistaken to assume I was holding back the danger myself.

It was something I had always done as a child. If I behave, my father might stop drinking. If I love him a little more. If I keep ballroom dancing with him into the late hours of the night. None of these things ever worked, of course, and yet I continued to carry the weight of trying to keep the peace in our home for many years.

It is one thing to say, I trust you God.

It is entirely different to walk and live in that trust.

My trust had to be in the character of who God was.

A God who is abounding in love and faithfulness and healing.

CHAPTER 11

RESTORATION AND HEALING

THE SPIRITUAL SWORD I was now learning to hold had a significant part to play in my healing. This new sword had to cut deeply at the base of the roots of any childhood wounds that were still influencing my life. I sought out a counsellor.

Not just any counsellor. I needed a counsellor that was a woman of faith; a counsellor that relied upon the counsellor Himself.

Isaiah 9:6 speaks of the many unique divine aspects of Jesus Himself:

> *For unto us a child is born, a son given to us.*
> *The government will rest upon his shoulders.*
> *And He will be called;*
> *Wonderful Counsellor, Mighty God, Everlasting Father, Prince of Peace.*

"Wonderful counsellor" speaks to us of a wisdom beyond human capabilities. It highlights the role of Jesus in guiding his followers through the complexities of life with divine wisdom.

Seeking a counsellor or trusted friend who is led by godly wisdom is important if you feel you need to pray through childhood wounds. It did not take long before I felt strongly directed to a past Christian friend who was a mentor to me some years earlier. She was located some 100 kilometers from my home. However, I knew it was the person God had placed before me. Every Wednesday night, as the children were heading to bed, I would begin the long drive to her home.

It was in this home where that spiritual sword laid bare my personal path to restoration and wholeness. We are all spirit, soul and body, and God is in the business of bringing wholeness not just to our physical body, but to our entire being. It was not easy to go back and acknowledge past wounds, and I am forever grateful to my friend and counsellor who went into battle with me… a counsellor who is still helping people find restoration in Jesus some 27 years later.

Together, we put the spiritual sword to the roots of unforgiveness, bitterness, and other parts of my life I needed to find freedom in.

Perhaps the most incredible part of my counselling journey was the prophetic bible verses given to me. Brave declarations over my future. A future I thought I may never have.

Time has in fact shown all those prophetic bible verses spoken over me to be accurate.

God gifted the extraordinary in the ordinary setting of my friend's home.

What I am about to say might sound somewhat controversial to some, but you do not need a church setting, corporate worship, or a special Christian conference to experience the power of God. No doubt these are important settings where God can move powerfully. If we look in the Bible however, Jesus performed many miracles for people in the most ordinary of places. There is no greater example of this than the woman at the well, who was simply drawing water, and met with the life changing, healing power of God.

If the woman at the well is not beyond God's miraculous reach, neither are we.

Now some may say we do not need to revisit past wounds or seek repentance for former things.

"We are a new creation in Christ", they declare. And I agree, we are. And yet, I believe salvation is only the first step in a lifetime of transformation in Jesus.

I was desperate for the abundant, whole, healed life Jesus' spoke of in the Bible. If you are reading this and you feel there are stumbling blocks in your own life, ask God to show you what they are, and pray through them. Get brave and bold before God. Pray and remove any hindrance between you and your loving Father.

A crucial truth, however, needs clarification at this point in my story.

Whenever I come alongside Christians who are in a battle with sickness, a disturbing narrative at times seems to emerge. This false narrative is often an underlying, unspoken burden they are unnecessarily carrying.

It is the burden of shame.

This burden is a lie.

Your sickness is not the result of anything you have done.

Let that sink deep down into your very soul. Yes, we are wise to seek freedom from past wounds, but sickness is never from the hand of a loving Father.

Sickness and shame have no place in a healthy relationship with a loving God.

What I am suggesting is that old wounds may lessen the fullness of the restoration and healing God so dearly wants to bring into our lives.

I am not suggesting the darkness of adversity you are facing is from the hand of the Lord. The Lord will, however, show up in your pain in good and wonderful and miraculous ways, if you let Him.

God revealed my personal path to healing as I stepped out and trusted Him.

My journey is not your journey.

My hope is that my journey may hold some spiritual truths to help you, as you courageously seek healing from God. Stay alert for shame and dismiss it from your mind immediately.

There is therefore now no condemnation to them which are in Christ Jesus, who walk not after the flesh, but after the spirit. (Romans 8:1)

CHAPTER 12

ENDURING VICTORIOUSLY

WE DO NOT GET stronger when we are unchallenged. Looking back on all the hard times in my life, I begrudgingly start to see a pattern emerging. I say "begrudgingly" because none of us like being in the valleys of life. We much prefer the mountain tops, where the view is clear and we can see the horizon. We know where we are heading.

The mountain top gives us a commanding view of the land surrounding us and what lies ahead. We feel safe there, in control, in command of our lives. A mountain climber arrives at the top of a mountain with victory in his heart and soul after an arduous and dangerous journey. And yet, once the mountain has been climbed, it has been conquered.

Invariably, there is always another mountain that comes into view on the not-too-distant horizon. It is, however, the valleys that in fact lead us toward the next mountain top.

Last spring, my husband and I had the incredible experience of walking in the French Alps. Coming from Australia, everything was so vastly different. The mountains held a grandeur that was so breathtaking. The sunrises arrived much later, and there seemed to be a long pause as we waited for first light to creep over the nearest mountain peak.

We walked beside mountain creeks, where the flowing water brought an immeasurable sense of peace.

It was God's creation in its finest glory.

One day, as we wandered through a valley with steep mountains either side, I noticed how the valley was carving out which way to walk, and the mountains themselves were shielding us from the strong winds forecast for the day. I suddenly felt the closeness of God as we walked, almost hemmed in by His creation and His goodness.

It seemed strange to feel the protective closeness of God as I walked in this literal valley because previously, I had always viewed valleys in a negative way.

In the Bible, valleys are often a metaphor for difficult times; times of darkness and despair, defeat, or discouragement.

The valleys of our life can be used by God to create a stronger faith in us, if we bravely allow Him to.

A stronger, intimate closeness with Him can be found.

A stronger knowledge, that he is with us, always.

There are spiritual nuggets of gold scattered through the valleys, even though the pain at times is unbearable.

These nuggets of gold will weave into our personal faith story, a story that will inevitably bring comfort and hope to others.

Even though I walk through the darkest valley, I will fear no evil, for you are with me. (Psalm 23:4)

I have also come to understand and respectfully value that a healing journey can look like a season where you, or someone you love, is enduring victoriously.

A dear friend, who is in a health battle as I am writing my story, graciously shared this personal scripture that encouraged her greatly.

If troubles weigh you down, that just means that we receive even more comfort to pass on to you for your deliverance! For the comfort pouring into us empowers us to bring comfort to you. And with this comfort upholding you, you can endure victoriously the same suffering we experience. (2 Corinthians 1:2)

Enduring victoriously.

What a powerful posture of faith as a believer.

Not just enduring, but enduring with hope.

Not just enduring, but enduring in His strength.

Not just enduring, but finding Jesus in the intimate detail of whatever adversity you are facing.

Not just enduring, but seeing glimpses of the goodness of God in the middle of our pain.

Glimpses of the goodness of God can help sustain us through the seemingly unexplainably tough parts of our journey. When my mum was in her battle against cancer, I saw many instances of the goodness of God that covered and protected her from some of the difficult things along the way.

Nausea from treatment lifted. Expected side effects were minimal. Energy to interact with her grandchildren remained. The wisdom of doctors leading her to make medical decisions that were favourable.

Above all, an unexplainable faith and joy that lifted her above her circumstances.

My mother chose life, despite her sickness.

She chose hope, instead of fear and anxiety. She chose to meditate on the healing words of Jesus, rather than the negative words of the medical report.

Can I encourage you to not just see healing as an end point, but rather, to look for small evidences of God's miracles along the way.

Jesus is always interceding on our behalf and contending for wholeness for you. Jesus hates sickness as much as we do.

Look for Him in your battle. You will find him standing with you.

Look for His miracles of mercy along the way.

Looking for the evidence of God, will bring you great courage, as you keep moving forward.

Healing can take time.

Our youngest son, was born with a lung condition that emerged at four weeks of age.

He was tested for Cystic Fibrosis as a baby and the test was negative. The test would be repeated twice more by various specialists throughout his early childhood with the final one at eight years of age. A bronchoscopy was also performed and the doctors were troubled by the huge amount of sticky mucous in his bronchial passages.

There was no clear diagnosis for why his lungs were filling with mucous. He may not have tested positive to CF, but he displayed all the symptoms of the disease. He was thin and pale and spent most nights sleeping in our bed, where we could easily lay him over the edge of our bed and thump his back, using a physio technique we had learned to help clear his lungs.

I am sharing this story with you to build your hope if you have been in a health battle for a long period of time.

Never give up.

Keep persisting in prayer even when you are stumbling around in the darkness of a circumstance you do not fully understand.

We prayed for twelve years and eventually the natural world gave way to the spiritual world.

Was it hard? Absolutely heartbreaking at times.

Why did it take 12 long years for my beautiful boy to be healed?

I do not know.

What I do know, is that God is faithful and He hears every heartfelt prayer, as we stand bravely in the hard, waiting and trusting Him.

Our twelve-year-old sickly boy with an undiagnosed lung condition is now inexplicably healed, with a perfectly working set of lungs.

He has grown up to be a God gifted musician, singing and writing worship songs for Jesus.

So, lift your hands and thank God for His marvellous kindness and for all His miracles of mercy for those He loves. (Psalm 107 v 8 TPT)

Walking with anguish does not mean a lack of faith in God.

The unwanted heavy burden of anguish can ultimately become a gift in our lives.

CHAPTER 13

ANGUISH IN YOUR SOUL

DO NOT BE AFRAID of the times in life when you may experience deep anguish in your soul.

Walking with anguish does not mean a lack of faith in God.

In the book of Isaiah, the King of Judah, Hezekiah, speaks of a deep anguish in his soul when he was struggling with illness. He refers to this anguish as the very thing that kept him walking humbly under the hand of God.

Anguish can be an unwanted burden that can ultimately become a gift in our lives.

> *I will walk humbly all my years because of the anguish in my soul*
> *Lord, by such thing's men live; and my spirit finds life in them too.*
> *You restored me to health and let me live.*
> *Surely it was for my benefit that I suffered such anguish. (Isaiah 38 v 15 -17)*

If you are walking with deep anguish in your soul today, God understands.

Jesus himself felt unimaginable anguish as the time drew closer to his crucifixion.

In the garden of Gethsemane, he cried out to God. You may not understand the purpose of the adversity you have found yourself in, and yet, in due time, with hindsight and understanding, the anguish in our lives can become a sacred part of our personal faith story.

Every year, before I enter the doctor's office for my annual checkup, my anguish rises. God, however, understands the anguish that we carry. The anguish of the what-ifs; the anguish of what if God takes His healing hand off my disease?

The anguish of what if I am not here to see my young children grown?

Why has God left the myeloma markers in my blood? He is more than capable of removing them from my blood test.

I believe it has been the very thing that has kept me walking closely to Him.

What was meant for evil, He has turned for good.

The anguish that has accompanied me has in fact transformed me.

The deep anguish has, in fact, become a gift to me also, just like Hezekiah. A gift that has been the very thing that has shown me, right up close, how to walk by faith.

I walk humbly by faith because it is only through the power of a mighty God that my disease has remained stable.

I walk humbly by faith because I am a miracle that has confounded the doctors.

I walk humbly by faith because my healing is nothing of me, and all of Him.

Many years ago, a scripture verse was given to me personally and it became an anchor of hope for me; a verse that has proven to be a prophetic declaration over my life, as each year has passed.

> *This sickness will not end in death.*
> *No, it is for God's glory so that Gods son may be glorified through it (John 11.4)*

Walking humbly even despite the anguish that rises from time to time, has become an ever-grateful natural posture for me.

It has now been 27 years since my diagnosis, and I think I may have finally begun to grasp perhaps part of the reason I am still here.

I am not here for me.

I am here for Him.

I am here to give God the glory.

I cry every birthday. In fact, not just on my birthday.

I tend to cry at every milestone that marks the passing of time. I cry because it is a miracle that I am still here.

I cry because my heart becomes overwhelmed by the goodness of God and because I must admit that this battle has left behind a certain level of grief in my life.

I will admit that the shadow of the diagnosis has undoubtedly stolen some of my joy at times.

I cry with tears of joy however, because this young mother has now seen both her sons fully grown.

A milestone that I thought was never possible.

Even before my health challenge, I had always found birthdays emotional to celebrate. Perhaps my response had been shaped by birthdays past, birthdays shrouded in fear and disappointment during my childhood. I recall as a young girl turning 13 and moving into my teenage years, all I wanted was one thing: the miracle of a father who would arrive at my teenage birthday dinner, sober. I prayed and pleaded with God that He would help my father come to my celebration sober.

Just this once. Just for me. It was a gift I had longed for my whole childhood.

And yet, sadly, my father would not find the courage to stop using alcohol on that day.

He staggered into my birthday dinner and as he headed straight for the bar, my teenage hopes were once again destroyed and the false idea that God could not hear my prayers had slowly taken hold.

I cried on my 13th birthday.

I cried on my recent 63rd birthday.

The cry, however, is now totally different. God has transformed my tears.

The tears that were once of great sadness and utter fear, have been miraculously changed into tears of hope.

They are now the tears of a grateful heart that cannot fathom the miracle-working power of God in my life.

They are now tears of trust in a loving God.

God was not like my earthly father after all.

"Let the redeemed of
the Lord tell their story,
those He redeemed from
the hand of the foe."

                    Psalm 107:1-2

CHAPTER 14

LET THE REDEEMED TELL THEIR STORY

Give thanks to the Lord, for he is good;
His love endures forever.
Let the redeemed of the Lord tell their story,
those he redeemed from the hand of the foe. (Psalm 107 v 1.2)

"LET THE REDEEMED OF the Lord tell their story, those he redeemed from the hand of the foe."

This is the very reason I have chosen to share my story. The Lord did redeem my life from the hand of the foe.

The foe can be many things. The foe is whatever mountain of adversity you are facing today. Anxiety, depression, loss, grief, illness.

Nothing is too far from the outstretched Hand of God.

No adversity is too hard for Him.

As I shared earlier, I am writing my story some 27 years since my initial diagnosis of multiple myeloma. I am now a mother and a grandmother.

The specialist now refers to my disease as smoldering multiple myeloma, since it has remained unexpectedly stable for such a long period of time, and I have not required any treatment. Every year, the blood test to check on my myeloma challenges my faith immensely. In complete honesty, every year, I battle the same demons: doubt, fear, unbelief.

Every year, the myeloma cells are still showing in my blood test, as well as other markers of its presence, and the doctor reminds me of the very real risk of my myeloma progressing to active disease.

Every year, however, my doctor seems a little confounded.

I am a patient sitting outside the realm of his medical statistics, an outlier of sorts.

I am a patient who challenges his scientific view of disease, and while I hold the utmost respect for the discipline of medicine, it should not in itself disqualify God's sovereign Hand in our lives.

Worldly wisdom from God's perspective, was at times a stumbling block to belief.

There were instances where Jesus challenged the intellectual path to finding faith as one that can be fraught with unbelief.

I will dismantle the wisdom of the wise and I will invalidate the intelligence of the scholars.

(I Corinthians 1.29.TPT)

So, every year, I respectfully remind my doctor of something too.

I remind him I have been praying and trusting God with my life. He always looks uncomfortable as God has perhaps been "*dismantling his wisdom*" over the years. He does, however, say the same response back to me. "Well, just keep doing what you are doing, it is working."

God's prognosis has well and truly surpassed the doctor's report all those years ago, spoken over this young mother.

God is a sovereign Father and each one of us is an individual, created in His image.

Each one, called for His purposes. Each one, called by name.

Each one, called home on the day only He determines.

> *My frame was not hidden from you when I was made in the secret place.*
> *When I was woven together in the depths of the earth, your eyes saw my unformed body.*
> *All the days ordained for me, were written in your book before one of them came to be. (Psalm 139 v15-16)*

I have had to learn to walk a journey of faith, where I have had to choose the healing words of Jesus as the framework of Truth for my life.

Let me conclude my story by returning to our incredible sons, who continue to be the greatest gift to me. They are both married now to strong women of faith and have young children of their own.

My husband and I held my diagnosis closely for some 20 years before we eventually felt God was prompting us to tell our grown sons. I felt a strong conviction around not holding it as a secret anymore, as I was now withholding a miracle from them.

I was withholding the glory that rightfully belonged to God.

It was time.

Time to reveal the miracle of God that had preserved my life, preserved their mother, and forever changed the course of our entire family.

My hope is that as their lives unfold, they will be eternally grateful for a God who is faithful through the generations.

A God who they know beyond a doubt, they can trust wholeheartedly.

A God who can bring life to dead bones.

A God who can bring flooding water to dry places in their lives.

A God who will be with them, in the inevitable valleys that will come.

A God who can perform miracles.

My hope for you, too, is that you can bravely choose faith in God over fear, regardless of whatever mountain of adversity you are facing.

That you choose to anchor your hope in a God who I have personally discovered to be a more than trustworthy foundation.

A God who is abounding in goodness, faithful to His promises, and is fully capable of performing *miracles of mercy and healing* in your life.

Jesus Christ the Saviour is still healing and holding back disease today.

I understand the daily struggle it is to trust in Him completely.

But this I can assure you:

That choosing to dwell in a place of healing and hope with Jesus, will always be the most loved, protected, and victorious place to stand.

Stand defiantly with God in the darkness, light your candle and declare;

"I beg to differ."

> *Generation after generation stands in awe of your work;*
> *Each one tells stories of your mighty acts.*
> *Your beauty and splendour have everyone talking;*
> *I compose songs on your wonders.*
> *Your marvellous doings are headline news;*
> *I could write a book full of the details of your greatness. (Psalm 145:4-6 MSG)*

FAITH IN GOD

Faith in God is like climbing a mountain,
A little at a time,
At first the top seems out of reach,
But you must choose to begin the climb,
Faith is a decision.

After climbing some, you tire,
A plateau appears.
Faith is resting in Him.

As you continue the climb,
You grow weary
of the constant uphill struggle.
Faith is persistence.

You press on,
Seeking your pathway to the top.
Faith is really knowing and hearing from God.

Your foot slips on the slippery surface,
You reach for a firm rock nearby.
Faith is standing alongside others.

I BEG TO DIFFER

You keep climbing, regardless of the onlookers
at the bottom of the mountain,
who think you will never make it
Faith is a personal gift from God.

You look back to see how far you have come.
The view is magnificent.
Faith is joy and hope.

Keep on, as the top draws near,
Your loving Father yearns
to reward your steadfast faith in Him.
Faith is victory.

Susan Lambert 1998

ABOUT THE AUTHOR

Susan Lambert is a wife, mother and educator who lives with her husband in a small Australian coastal community, near the Pacific Ocean in Northern NSW. Her greatest fulfilment has been found in being the mother of two grown sons and more recently becoming a grandmother. *I Beg to Differ* is her second book.

susanlambertauthor.com

www.ingramcontent.com/pod-product-compliance
Lightning Source LLC
Chambersburg PA
CBHW020546080526
44583CB00013B/1018